KIDNEY FOR SALE

A struggle for survival

Yasmin Ghurki

Twenty five percent of profits from the sale of this book will go to Kidney Research UK; the leading national charity dedicated to research that will lead to better treatments and cures for kidney disease.

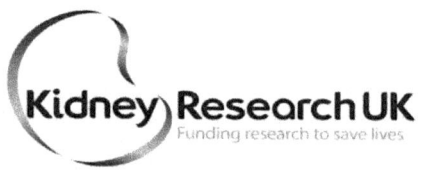

For more information and donations:

http://www.kidneyresearchuk.org/

Copyright © 2015 Yasmin Ghurki

Print Edition

ALL RIGHTS RESERVED. Any unauthorized reprint or use of this material is prohibited. No part of this book may be reproduced, or transmitted in any form or by any means, electronic or mechanical, including photocopying, recording, or by any information storage and retrieval system without express written permission from the author.

Disclaimer

Some names and identifying details have been changed to protect the privacy of individuals.

ISBN: 978-0-9956520-1-9

DEDICATION

Dedicated to my brother Asif, and all who are affected by kidney disease for their strength.

To all those families who have donated their loved ones organs under difficult situations to improve lives of others.

To those who are prepared to give a gift of life after their own death and have signed the organ donor register.

To join the organ donor register:

https://www.organdonation.nhs.uk/how_to_become_a_donor/registration/consent.asp

Contents

Dedication	4
Foreword	6
Chapter 1: Beat the Odds	7
Chapter 2: Not a Myth	14
Chapter 3: To Stay Alive	17
Chapter 4: In the Third World	21
Chapter 5: The Illegal Kidney Trade	25
Chapter 6: Kidney Buyers	28
Chapter 7: Kidney Sellers	31
Chapter 8: Playing the Game	35
Chapter 9: Out of Luck	41
Chapter 10: Hope for the Future	46
Disclaimer	51
Acknowledgements	52
A Note from Yasmin Ghurki	53

Foreword

This poignant account of Asif's battle with kidney disease highlights the desperation faced by many kidney patients across the world.

I would encourage everybody who reads this story to sign the organ donor register, but also to have a conversation with your own loved ones and family members so they know your wishes.

Only by having these conversations can we ensure that more donated organs are available in the UK, and more patients receive a transplant they need so desperately.

Thank you for your support.

Peter Storey

Director of Communications, Kidney Research UK.

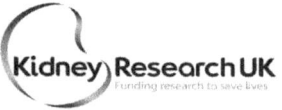

CHAPTER 1.
Beat the Odds

'I want to buy a kidney and I want you to help me.'

I will never forget my younger brother's words, spoken to me on New Year's Day, in 2007.' He had come especially to visit me at my home, and stood before me, utterly convinced of his decision.

My initial reaction to Asif's uncommon request was, "Are you serious?" Because it was not as though he wanted to buy a second-hand DVD set, or even a used car that we could just order off the Internet. As far as I knew, buying or selling a kidney was illegal in nearly all countries around the world. And why would he want to buy a kidney instead of waiting for a legitimate kidney donor?

The many TV documentaries I had watched over the years debating the ethics of the harvesting and selling of human body parts had long since made me discount this supposed 'option'. It was undoubtedly immoral to take part in this unthinkable proposition. Surely he should count his lucky stars that he was still alive? What a ludicrous idea!

But my brother was adamant, even though the doctors that had been treating him for years, advised him wholeheartedly against this plan. Patiently, they had explained the many, many associated risks to which he would be exposed. Still, with or without me, and without the support of his doctors, Asif was determined to follow his plan. It was my turn to think long and hard.

Asif was only five years old when his battle with kidney disease began. He was taken into hospital for a routine check-up but within weeks he lost his basic bodily functions, his ability to speak and his hearing.

Both of his kidneys failed, meaning his blood could no longer be naturally purified of nitrogenous waste products, and his body's fluid and ion levels could no longer be maintained without artificial assistance. Placed on a life support machine to be stabilized, he lay in a coma-like state for about three months.

The outlook was not good. As a last hope the doctors tried a new drug. It worked beyond all expectations, and not only was Asif able to come off the life support machine but both of his kidneys started functioning again and he regained the ability to communicate. The doctors could not explain what had happened. It was not something they had ever witnessed before and was an exceptionally rare case.

My parents and indeed our entire community – who had been praying for Asif – believed this to be nothing short of a miracle. After months of rehabilitation Asif was in good form.

In the years to follow, the function of Asif's kidneys gradually decreased and he had to take different medications and undergo many onerous operations. Until finally his kidneys both failed in 2000 and he began his journey with dialysis treatment.

Asif had to adapt quickly to dialysis. He took it on board with strength of mind though he knew it was not going to be an easy ride. It was Asif who had to make a long term plan with dialysis as part of his life and yet it affected all of us in the family.

We anticipated a transplant to take place in some years to come. But to our surprise our prayers were answered once again. After only dialyzing for a month Asif received a kidney from the donor pool. Instantly Asif's quality of life improved. He was able to enjoy his food and drinks and have a decent night's sleep. He resumed his studies and was filled with hope for the future. He was always grateful to the donor who gave him another chance.

Asif's donated kidney was from a cadaver or after death patient. Usually cadavers are expected to last up to twelve years but for Asif it only lasted for five years. There was no compatible donor from the family due to age, ill health and other obstacles. It was assured that Asif was on dialysis and on the waitlist. For most of Asif's life he never complained and just got on with living. However, after continuously dialyzing for nearly two years and his body taking its toll of pain my brother decided that he wanted a change for the better. My brother was in his twenties and wanted to experience what others his age readily took for granted.

Now a better life for some may mean more money, or a bigger house. Many seek to find a long-term companion or come to terms with their spirituality. Still others aim to achieve career aspirations or their deep-seated ambitions. For someone with kidney failure, a better life is simply the ability to live normally, without an existence revolving around hospital visits.

As with my brother, the only lifeline for most people with kidney failure is dialysis and the interminable wait for a kidney to become available from the donor pool. These kidneys mainly originate from deceased donors, with only a small percentage coming from live donors. While the demand for kidneys has been increasing and the waiting lists getting longer, the supply of kidneys has not.

Although dialysis replicates the kidneys' function and filters blood to rid the body of harmful waste, extra salt and water, it cannot replace a kidney entirely and, in time, other complications arise. For someone with end stage renal disease like Asif, dialysis can, on average, add only ten years to your life expectancy. A kidney transplant would give you twice as long.

Asif was undergoing haemodialysis. For this he had a fistula: an artificial access to the blood stream whereby the artery from his heart was connected to a vein in his forearm. Into this a needle was inserted, which was attached by a tube to a dialysis machine. Blood was transferred from his body into the machine, which filtered out waste products and excess fluids. The filtered blood was then passed back into his body.

"It's like shock waves inside and your head is going to explode." Asif commented the first time he dialyzed.

He had three sessions a week, each lasting four hours. Including travel and waiting time it actually took up to seven hours per session. Apart from the repeated needles inserted to connect to the dialysis machine three times a week, he had to get used to the usual side effects of dialysis. He suffered with intense fatigue due to the ongoing repercussions of the dialysis on his body and the related stress and anxiety it brought.

He experienced severe cramps caused by his muscles reacting to the fluid loss that occurs during haemodialysis. Also he experienced itchy skin due to a build-up of potassium in his body. He felt dizzy and sick to his stomach, and had difficulty both falling and staying asleep. He spent many a night sleeping in an upright position. He suffered bone and joint pain, and a dry mouth.

Asif had to take numerous medications to treat various ailments caused by renal failure. Amongst these were treatment for hypertension, low calcium, anaemia, heart and blood vessel disease. Not only that, he had to give up many foods and drinks that he loved. The freedom to travel just anywhere was soon a thing of the past as he was forced to plan his trips with dialysis mapped in; otherwise he simply could not go.

Yes, he was still alive, but I realised what haemodialysis did to him. He had to sleep for hours on end to recover and was subjected to heaps of other complications. There are many thousands of people all around the world like my brother affected by kidney failure and the figures are astounding. It can happen to any of us.

According to the UK's Special Health Authority; NHS Blood and Transplant (NHSBT), in the UK alone there are 10,000 patients who need new organs. Most commonly these are livers, kidneys and hearts. Each day three people die while waiting for a transplant.

People from Black, Asian and some minority ethnic communities are five times more likely to require organ transplantation as we are prone to illnesses such as diabetes, hypertension and hepatitis. The NHSBT reveals that at the end of March 2014, three out of ten patients on the kidney transplant list were from our communities. However, a staggering 66% of our communities in the UK refuse to give permission for our loved ones' organs to be donated. This is mainly due to lack of information available and certain religious beliefs that organ donation is forbidden as you have to return to the Maker as a whole.

There are simply not enough organs to meet demand, despite the demand continuing to rise. This situation is not limited solely to the UK – it is echoed around the world. There are many factors contributing to this issue, such as an overall increase in life expectancy, obesity and other lifestyle changes including higher alcohol consumption, all contributing to an increase in diseases such as diabetes, hypertension and hepatitis C.

Data from the World Health Organisation (WHO) shows that of all the solid organs transplanted in 2010 around the world, both legally and illegally, 68.5% were estimated to be kidneys. And that only satisfied 10% of the global demand.

Asif could wait for a kidney donor, and could get lucky again but the odds were similar to winning the lottery. On average, the wait for a kidney is three years in the UK. Since organs are matched best from one's own ethnic group and Asif was a British Pakistani, for him the wait was even longer.

In the UK, Black and Asian people face waiting for an average five years on dialysis, due to so few organ donations from our communities. In turn the longer term dialysis gives rise to other diseases which contribute to the reduction in life expectancy. Therefore people from our communities are more likely to die while waiting for a renal transplant.

Asif did not want to take the chance of becoming a statistic.

I realised his proposal was not that ludicrous after all. Right or wrong, I decided to help him.

Chapter 2

Not a Myth

The search for a kidney did not take as long as we had anticipated. In fact, in only a matter of days we found ways of acquiring one.

Just for curiosity's sake we typed 'kidney for sale' into Google and, to our surprise, a whole host of websites popped up offering the organ. So it was true you could buy anything off the Internet – not just books, clothes or electronic stuff!

Desperation was displayed throughout. From those who were in dire need of money and trying to sell their organ to those who were in dire need of a kidney and wanted to buy one due to the lack of donor organs available. There were plenty of agents who could assist in making it all possible at various hospitals in different parts of the world.

We contacted a few of these agents to find out more details. Deliberately, we chose agents in Pakistan and India due to Asif's ethnic background, therefore increasing the level of compatibility and potential success for a transplant, although the awareness of language and culture also played a big part. To be honest, had the kidney been available in any country at that point in time, Asif would have gone anywhere.

The response was promptly received from the agents, outlining all the details regarding the procedure of the sale, price, the people involved, and where it would take place. I remember laughing that, despite the fact that these agents were working in the black market, each still had a marketing plan – the 4 P's of the kidney market: Procedure, Price, People and Place! But it was not a laughing matter. Large sums of money, was involved in the black market for kidneys – no wonder there were so many agents facilitating sales. There were some who asked for a reasonable amount, while others were asking for a price of a house in a nice suburb of Manchester, in cash! The prices ranged from £15,000 to £250,000.

Well, we wanted to buy a kidney but we were not rich, with a lot of money to spare. Our mother – bless her – could not stand seeing Asif in any more pain and would have given anything for him to lead a normal life, get married and have kids. We are talking about her life savings here, which, needless to say, did not amount to anywhere near a nice suburban semi!

We set all the information before us and had to decide which of the agents to choose. Obviously at this point we were supremely anxious. The risks about which the hospital had warned Asif were real and we had to avoid these at all costs. There were many cases where patients had kidney transplants in these countries but on their return their new kidney stopped working due to low compatibility. Furthermore, a large number had caught other blood borne diseases and for some it was fatal.

While we were still deciding, luckily for us, only a few streets away from where my brother lived, someone our mother knew had just returned from Pakistan, having just purchased a kidney for her daughter. It was a real case and was exactly what we were hoping for. The daughter looked in great health and had been given the all clear from the hospital at which she previously dialysed in Manchester. So what had made them follow this illegal and a widely viewed 'unethical' option?

As far as the parents were concerned, dialysis was no life for their daughter. She was deteriorating on a daily basis and they simply could not see her face the misery of haemodialysis any longer. Without this kidney, the daughter would not have been sitting before us that day. Whilst we were at their house we were able to speak with Dr Akhtar, who had made the arrangements for their daughter's new kidney. He explained some of the details and the rest we had to follow up via email.

With a sigh of relief that we did not have to venture into totally unknown territory, we arranged to buy a kidney for Asif in Lahore, Pakistan. Not only did the doctors, hospitals and procedure seem safe, but we also had family there.

CHAPTER 3
To Stay Alive

In pursuit of a 'normal' life, one without having to rely on a dialysis machine to stay alive, Asif made his first trip to Lahore in January 2007. Our Mother accompanied him but I was unable to due to work commitments.

On this occasion Asif was not able to buy a kidney as his own defective kidneys had to be taken out first so that the new kidney would not be rejected. To do this a major operation was required, which carried many risks. However this did not worry Asif, since over the years he has had many operations and his body was full of evidence with stitch marks. He decided to have the surgery in Lahore without hesitation.

Just a week after his operation and with his wound still in stitches he came back home! Asif was advised to return for his new kidney once he had healed properly.

Four months later Asif made the second journey to Lahore. Mum and I went with him to help in his endeavour.

As soon as we arrived in Pakistan we arranged to meet Dr Akhtar at his clinic. We did not want to remain in Pakistan any longer than necessary as it was already proving to be a costly affair.

Our ride to the clinic was a rickshaw. Asif and I

had not been on one before! We slid into one without warning! The rickshaw zigzagged around other vehicles to get out ahead of the jammed roads, and just about missed the oncoming traffic. It flew over the bumps and flung us around! Luckily, after over an hour we arrived to our destination, in one piece!

The clinic was on one of Lahore's major roads. A long stretch of hospitals, offices, retail shops, hotels, restaurants and to our delight KFC and McDonalds!

We walked past the queue formed in the sweltering heat outside of the clinic, with all eyes on us. We nudged our way into the clinic already crammed with people. It was like a steam room. No air! Forget the conditioning!

Asif and I were ushered into Dr Akhtar's room straightaway. As he had dealt with Asif before, there was no need to assess if this was a genuine case. There was no worry of us being sent by an investigating body from the West, posing as patients!

Dr Akhtar was shorter than I had imagined him to be. He was dressed smartly with a shirt and tie and when he spoke English, he had an American accent! He had a bold and presumptuous manner, and yet he was likeable!

Dr Akhtar waved his hands around stressing that his clinic only did these operations to help people like Asif and that the money did not matter. It was like a favour – a social service rather than a financial greed – and that people should be grateful that the consultant, Dr Zaman actually did the operations at all. There was 'nothing immoral' about it, he said. He explained that Dr Zaman could just as easily go back to Canada and earn more money there than he would ever need!

Dr Akhtar's name may have been spelt differently but he certainly was an actor! We nodded our heads to show our gratitude. At this point we would have agreed to anything, because we were only interested in obtaining a kidney for Asif. If he had said that he was, in fact, Mother Teresa, we would have nodded and agreed!

Dr Zaman checked Asif out and advised that he was fit to have his operation. There were donors lined up already! Just a few final tests needed doing in their laboratory.

"It's just straight forward and nothing to worry about!" reassured Dr Zaman. Asif gave his blood samples, and took all the instructions. We left the clinic content that in a matter of days our mission would be accomplished.

We woke up the following morning to see the news. A group of poor labourers had been picked up in a truck supposedly bound for employment, but were later found dumped in an area just outside Lahore. Although they were still alive, each of the ten men had one of their kidneys removed without their knowledge or consent.

The news report went on to say that this was clearly part of an organised crime ring, with top doctors and hospitals forming the black market kidney trade in Pakistan. How could society have stooped to this despicable level?

Under considerable international pressure, the Pakistani government immediately banned kidney transplants for all patients, and definitely no foreigners would be permitted transplants until the case was heard by the High Court.

It dawned on us that we were foreigners too! Here we were, thousands of miles away from home, and trying to do something that did not feel quite right anymore.

"We only buy kidneys from donors who give their consent, No others. It's not a crime to do that." said Dr Akhtar defending his clinic and making it all normal.

In a sense it was not a crime because there was no other way that people could get a kidney in Pakistan. They did not have a donor register as in the UK or other western countries. If there were no relatives who were suitable donors then they had to buy kidneys. So there had to be sellers. Otherwise more people would die. It was widely accepted in Pakistan.

Dr Akhtar advised us to wait, as it would be only a few weeks before the case was heard and then the ban would no doubt be lifted. We had placed our trust in him and decided to wait for a few weeks.

In the meantime, Asif would have his dialysis done at an associate dialysis clinic.

Chapter 4.
In the Third World

The dialysis clinic was a hired room on the second floor within another hospital not far from the main clinic on the same road. A couple of men, wearing blue hospital uniforms walked around attending to people.

Asif checked in at the desk and handed over the saline and other dialysis medicines which we had purchased from the hospital chemist. He had to wait for ten minutes as the dialysis machine was being cleaned.

A dozen beds piled next to each other. On them people of different ages attached to dialysis machines with blood running in and out of their bodies through plastic tubes. Some of them snored away, whilst others chatted with their relatives sitting beside them chomping on food!

Asif lay on his bed connected to a machine. I tried to get comfy on a plastic chair for the next four hours!

On the opposite side a patient finished his dialysis, the bed sheet was just straightened out and one of the staff pressed some buttons to set the machine to clean and supposedly sterilise it for the next user. After ten minutes the bed and machine were taken again. Over the hours we noticed the people moving off and on beds. The beds were never empty for long. The machines switched users within fifteen minutes. This would happen on all our visits over the course of the months that Asif dialysed at this clinic.

We should have asked questions regarding the dialysis machines being cleaned properly as per industry standards. In truth, we were too overwhelmed by the devastating news events, the heat, and being in an unfamiliar environment – not to mention the anticipation of acquiring a kidney to save my brother.

To make matters worse, not all of the staff had proper credentials to work in a hospital or clinic. They must have simply been shown how to operate the machines as though in a factory!

On one occasion Asif knew his blood pressure was very high and asked to have it checked. He was told that his blood pressure was 120 over 80, which is normal, but Asif's blood pressure had not been anywhere near this for years! It can be fatal for a patient to have very high blood pressure during a dialysis session. After this, Asif insisted on always taking his own digital blood pressure machine wherever he went.

Asif needed three sessions a week of dialysis. Coming from the UK where we are lucky enough to get everything free through the National Health Service (NHS), we did not realise exactly how costly dialysis is. Back home, Asif qualified for a free taxi ride to and from routine hospital visits as well to attend dialysis sessions. He did not have to worry about things like obtaining medication or saline for the dialysis machine. The costs here were mounting up!

In Pakistan one session of dialysis alone costs more

than the average Pakistani earns in a month. If you are poor and your kidneys fail, you are simply told by the doctors that there is nothing that can be done and you face death in a matter of weeks. The rationalisation is that they cannot justify saving one person's life to the detriment of the rest of the family. In a place where people are struggling daily to put food on their plates, paying for dialysis would surely summon them all to their deaths.

We thought this was cruel but there was literally no other choice for these people. There is no NHS in Pakistan. Third world government hospitals cannot meet demand and are not able to provide this service on a free basis. There are other hospitals in the country that are run on charity money. These also cannot provide such a service for free. Unfortunately, for the majority of the population in Pakistan, dialysis will never be an affordable option.

Our visits at the dialysis clinic were like being in a regular soap opera! Most often we saw the same faces and caught up with the events of the previous days. Checked out rumours and found out things we did not know!

We were shocked to learn that 'Dr' Akhtar was actually not a medical doctor but a nurse by trade. He was a key agent who facilitated all the buying and selling of kidneys for his clinic and many others.

The consultant physician, Dr Zaman had been medically trained in Canada, worked in a major Pakistani government hospital and was renowned in his field. He, together with Akhtar, owned both clinics; the latter running the rest of the ventures.

This clinic was a real moneymaking business. All the

people coming through the doors of the other clinic to see Dr Zaman, and could afford it, were referred here for their dialysis. If there were not enough beds, then the rest were sent elsewhere in other hospitals, with Akhtar receiving a cut of the dialysis profits.

Akhtar turned out to be a very shrewd businessman. As well as these clinics he ran a successful brokering of kidneys.

CHAPTER 5
The Illegal Kidney Trade

Akhtar was a major player in Pakistan's black market kidney trade. We could never have guessed!

"He's a sly fox." said, one of the staff members at the clinic.

Akhtar's experience and connections in the medical field meant that he could easily arrange the operations. He had access to top medical people, hospitals and equipment. He was in a perfect position to facilitate the illegal kidney trade.

Akhtar was part of a larger network made up of a widely distributed group of people. It had connections not only in Pakistan but around the world. One of the many branches of the system linked back to Akhtar.

Akhtar had a key role in all transactions taking place. He arranged all the medical tests for the buyers and sellers. He sorted the medical personnel, hospitals, and operation schedules. He was the one who handled the money matters; paying the commissions and setting the price.

The illegal kidney trade conjured up hideous images of operations happening in unknown places resembling more butchers' shops than medical environments. This was far from the truth. Illegal though it was; operations were undertaken in hospitals by medical teams with high credentials.

Akhtar used the main clinic as the centre of the buying and selling activities. Renal failure patients from all over Pakistan attended the clinic to seek help from Dr Zaman. A large percentage of these attended due to referrals made by other doctors and hospitals receiving commission from Akhtar. This was not solely limited to Pakistan. The Agents targeted renal centres in other countries with offers of commission to the medical personnel and renal patients to market to other patients.

Akhtar and his network used the internet and social media sites to run their operation. They used this from attracting buyers in all corners of the globe, to enticing people to sell their kidneys in remote villages of Pakistan.

All the buyers and sellers were passed onto Akhtar to negotiate the deal. It is at this stage the sellers give their consent, just like Akhtar had said to us.

We were able to obtain all the information regarding Akhtar's business activities in such a short time. How come the authorities did not see any of it?

Akhtar had such a solid system in place that these clinics had never fallen under scrutiny from the authorities.

"Akhtar plays the game well and won't let anything spoil it." Our Source tells us.

He was protected by people in high places and the police. They had been paid off by him, so they turned a blind eye!

Since the media was actively reporting on the issues

surrounding kidneys and the ban, Akhtar had to halt activities at his clinics to keep them out of the limelight. But there was nothing stopping him from carrying on elsewhere without anyone's knowledge!

Chapter 6
Kidney Buyers

Asif and I met many different people at the dialysis clinic, all with their own individual stories. Amongst these were several foreigners, each one more desperate than the last.

There was an Arab millionaire who wanted to buy a kidney for his wife. He came to Pakistan as there were no kidneys available in his country, even though money was no object to him. He had heard from the hospital in Saudi Arabia that there were plenty of kidneys in Pakistan! He arrived only to find the ban in place. After waiting for several weeks they went back home with a view to return to Pakistan once everything settled down.

A Nigerian businessman was there in the hope of saving his elderly mother, whose dialysis was making her horribly ill. They arrived about a week before us and everything had been scheduled for a kidney transplant but then the ban came into effect. They too decided to wait like us, and we all often bumped into each other at the dialysis clinic.

Two American parents and their teenage son also arrived a week earlier. They were not rich – just your average income family – but, like my mum, willing to spend their entire savings so that their son could have a better quality of life with more years added on. After a week we no longer saw them, and rumour had it that Akhtar had sent them to another hospital where some kidney transplants, were still taking place. This hospital most likely bribed people in higher places to protect them from being investigated.

We were told that we were just a small number of foreigners being dealt with by Akhtar and his team, many more had come before us and there were always people in waiting. Besides the foreigners, this clinic seemed to have no shortage of domestic customers either, some who could just about afford the dialysis and others looking to buy a kidney.

We often saw a local man in his late forties accompanied by his wife. His groans whilst having dialysis grabbed everyone's attention. It was like someone was throttling him! His wife told me that their whole life had changed six months previously when her husband's kidneys failed. They had three young children aged nine, five and three years. She no longer had much time with them as her time was taken up by her husband. They were left with their grandparents most of the time. Her husband owned a textile factory but with him being so ill, their business was suffering too. They came here because their doctor advised them that the best option was to have a transplant and referred them to Akhtar.

One young girl had been on dialysis for a few weeks. Just sixteen years of age, she was due to have a transplant, with the kidney donated by her maternal uncle. Unfortunately the stay order for all kidney transplants then came into play. The cost of waiting for the ban to lift and continuing her dialysis was placing an immense strain on her family finances and, as a consequence, she had to cease dialysis.

The family was under a lot of stress; it was supposed to be a straightforward case with expenses only for the operation. The decision of stopping dialysis would most definitely prove to be fatal but they no longer had enough money to pay for it.

Happily the girl's prayers were answered, because within days of stopping her dialysis the court lifted the ban from transplants carried out with kidneys donated from relatives. She had her new kidney successfully transplanted later that day.

But for the rest of us, it was not to be. Weeks passed and Akhtar still insisted for us to wait as a change was imminent. So we waited. To keep us keen and not leave, or perhaps to stop us from looking at alternatives, Akhtar told us that he had found a couple of donors that matched. While he did not want us to meet any donor, and everything was shrouded under a veil of secrecy, we managed to speak to some ourselves in Akhtar's own clinic.

Chapter 7
Kidney Sellers

We contacted Akhtar at least every other day to find out if things had changed. It came to a point that he did not have anything new to say and often his secretary told us that he was unavailable as he was in theatre, at another hospital, or had not yet arrived at the clinic. There were many, other such pretences. To catch him at the clinic, sometimes Asif and I visited uninvited.

Even though we were of Pakistani origin, spoke the language and wore traditional dress, people could tell we were not from Pakistan just by looking at us! Many a time on the way to Akhtar's clinic we were approached by various people wanting to sell their kidneys, as they believed all foreigners attending this clinic only come for one thing.

We were curious to discover what was driving these people to sell their body parts. So we spoke to a few of them to find out what their reasons were and what were they expecting to gain from such a transaction.

One day we spoke to a man named Ali, who was in his mid thirties. He came from a village outside of Lahore, where he lived with his extended family of twelve members. He was the sole breadwinner for the family and worked as a manual labourer, lifting heavy materials in the construction industry. His take home wage was two thousand Pakistani Rupees in a month, which was barely enough to feed the household.

Ali said he needed money for his younger sister's dowry, without which she would remain forever at home, unmarried. Their family honour was on the line. Hence he was here looking to sell his kidney. He had already spoken to Akhtar who promised him that he would receive about two hundred thousand rupees for his organ. He was grateful to Akhtar for this big amount; because now not only could his sister marry, but he could buy a few cows that would provide milk, some of which he could sell and the rest keep for the family's use.

At the time that amount converted to approximately £1,600. A measly sum, considering Akhtar was charging us around £26,000. We were very uncomfortable with the fact that the donor who provided the actual lifeline got such a tiny percentage of the fee. When we confronted Akhtar with this knowledge he did not even attempt to hide the truth and just replied that there was a long chain and high medical fees involved. He said the donors were aware of the price beforehand and had total autonomy with the decision. Plus he said we were also lucky to get that price, since our agreement the price had increased!

On another occasion we spoke to eighteen-year-old Hassan and his cousin, who had travelled a hundred miles from their village to Lahore. Their family had to pay off a big loan owed to a landowner. If they failed to do so they would lose their home and have nowhere else to go. They found out about the clinic through someone who had sold his kidney previously. Both cousins were planning to sell their kidneys, as selling only one would not provide a large enough return. They were expecting a similar amount to Ali per kidney. They seemed blissfully unaware of the risks that they were taking at such a young age.

We met a couple of female donors too. One was a mother who was looking to sell her kidney because she needed the money for hospital fees for her ill son. Another was a widow who needed the cash for basic upkeep of her children. We asked them if they knew the risks involved. What if things did not turn out as expected? Their response was plain and simple. There were no alternatives for them; kismet had brought them here, it was written in their destiny. No wonder Akhtar justified it as a kind of 'social service'!

It was clear to us that people were willing to risk their lives by selling their kidneys or any other body part to ensure the safety of their loved ones' futures. Poverty was the underlying factor that drove all the people that we spoke with to take desperate measures and sell their kidneys. They simply did not have the free will in the same way we did in the West. Their will was driven by their financial and economical situations. For some it was a choice between selling a kidney or let their children starve. For these and for hundreds of others we only ever hear about in the media, this was the only way out. It was the only thing that they owned of value that they could sell and the only glimmer of hope.

It was overwhelming. The whole scheme of things, the poverty, the trust in Akhtar to pay a fair price – their kismet and ours. But then Mum told us of her own experience of poverty, growing up in her rural village near Rawalpindi and how she had left her family and friends to come to England to secure a poverty-free life for us her children. She told us of the time when there were none of the modern facilities that we now take for granted, only the agricultural land and what was grown on it. To be part of our family was considered lucky; as our grandfather had plenty of land so could grow food and draw water from the wells. Many poor people would come and take produce from our grandfather's land just to get by, some resorting to stealing, and others gathering each tiny grain off the ground.

Mum told us of hungry children's cries heard through the nights, soaring higher than the mosques' loudspeaker systems. Poor mothers often pretended to cook on log fires, whilst their famished children drifted off to sleep. Nursing mothers did not produce enough milk for their babies. People scavenged through piles of rubbish in the fields. Mum told us how people were forced to do all sorts of things in order to get rid of hunger, unimaginable things. A life of poverty was one of coercion and if it meant selling a kidney, so be it.

Asif was no longer sure that he even wanted to buy a kidney. He did not want to be selfish and take advantage of these poverty-stricken people's despair. Nevertheless we convinced him to go through with it. Just as the poor were desperate to protect their loved ones, our family was desperate to safeguard Asif's health and future. If they were already in the kidney market to sell, then they would sell anyway because life forced them to. If not to him, they would sell it to someone else.

Chapter 8
Playing the Game

The Pakistani temperature soared to over 40°C, exacerbated by load shedding of electricity (an intentionally engineered electrical power shutdown) lasting for hours at a time. We were used to UK temperatures which, with some luck, may reach 25°C degrees centigrade during summertime.

Our anxiety grew as the days went by. Things had not gone according to plan. We waited for the court hearing, only to see it adjourned. Each time we decided to wait for the next one and time after time they were adjourned. There was no foreseeable end to our predicament. Days turned into weeks, into months!

When Akhtar realised that we would leave, and no money will come his way, he scrambled to find ways of fulfilling our need. At one stage he said as a 'favour' he was willing to go against the law to help us! With the knowledge of his activities we were not surprised!

Akhtar conjured up a scheme to manipulate the law. Since the law was now not banning transplants with relatives, he suggested we lie and pretend that the donor was a relative. He said the operation could be carried out undercover and quickly. By the time the law caught up with us, we would have left the country. Wrong as it may seem, we were actually ready to go along with it and only stopped when Akhtar told us that Dr Zaman, refused to carry out the operation because of the risk to his reputation!

The real reason was somewhat different according to our source. Akhtar must have decided that his idea was not worthwhile, as we posed a bigger risk of exposing his links. We were of Pakistani origin with family in the country unlike all the other foreigners where there was no come back.

By now we had been in Pakistan for well over two months and time was running out. We had already stretched our stay to the maximum of which our commitments back in the UK allowed. This forced us to explore other options, just the same as the other foreigners.

Word had got out for the reason of our long stay in Pakistan and anxious relatives tried to be of assistance. Our cousin Fiaz had experience of buying a kidney, having previously found a donor for his maternal uncle who lived in France. His uncle could not travel to Pakistan, so the donor, Shamu, was taken to him. To compensate Shamu for his time and effort, he was paid all the money in advance.

In France, as in all other European countries, it is illegal to buy and sell body parts. To by-pass this, Shamu posed as the son of a childhood friend, who wanted to give Fiaz's uncle his kidney altruistically because the uncle had supposedly been 'like a father' to him!

Before the transplant could take place, Shamu was obliged to participate in vigorous interviews and tests. He became anxious and had second thoughts about donating his kidney. Furthermore, something about his story did not add up and the hospital authorities turned him down. Coming perilously close to being investigated for illegal transaction, he was quickly dispatched back to Pakistan with an agreement that the operation would take place there.

Once in Pakistan, Shamu could not be located and appeared to have run away with the cash. After warnings were sent to his family, he came out of hiding and, because he no longer had all the money given to him by Fiaz's uncle, he agreed to go ahead with the donation. Shamu was given more money after the operation as a goodwill gesture for his troubles. The whole process took about a year-and-a-half and had undoubtedly been highly stressful, but the transplant was successful and had changed the uncle's life.

In order to find a suitable donor, Fiaz took us to Shamu's village. We soon realised why, as we met many of the residents who had previously donated their kidneys. We asked them if it had changed their lives for the better. Were they still happy with their decisions? The majority agreed that although they did not regret what they had done, the money did not last long. As expected, the agents had passed on only a small cut of the fee to these innocent donors. There was one man whose agent vanished. He never received payment. In comparison, Shamu had been well compensated for his kidney and appeared happy and healthy. He agreed to contact Fiaz when he found a donor for Asif.

Next, Fiaz introduced us to the doctor who had performed his uncle's operation. This hospital was in total contrast to Akhtar's setup. The dialysis was performed in a controlled, clean environment just the same as in any UK hospital, with only the patients and the medical teams allowed to be present during dialysis. In Akhtar's dialysis clinic, I always accompanied Asif, as did the other patients' families. At times we even sat there and ate our food! This doctor was willing to do the operation but not until the ban was lifted.

Meanwhile, another relative had found an agent who could source a donor and medical team in a different part of Pakistan, and in a well-respected hospital. The fee was higher but we were willing to pay that price and travel to the other side of Pakistan, as long as the transplant could take place. We had to wait until this agent had made all the necessary arrangements for the transplant and for him to contact us.

Back at the dialysis clinic, the Nigerian businessman told us that he was taking his mother to another hospital where they were still performing undercover transplants. He had already arranged for her operation. He seemed pretty content with this decision and convinced us to do likewise. His mum's operation was only a couple of days away so we took his contact details and waited to learn the outcome.

As it turned out, we did not have to wait for long. Soon this hospital was also in the news and under police investigation. The police believed that a body, which had been found dumped in another place, was that of a kidney donor who tragically died on the operating table at this very hospital. The doctors and owners of the hospital had fled and were in hiding. To think we were considering putting all our hope and faith in these people!

One day Asif and I went to Lahore's Liberty market to buy some toiletries. Whizzing sounds of horns, traffic of vehicles and people filled the air. Cars, rickshaws, bicycles, people driven carriages, donkey driven carriages and a few others blocked the entrance!

As we shoved through the crowd we came to a trench like building works area. I jumped over this long deep hole with steep concrete sides and my feet landed safely across it. I heard a big thud behind me and when I turned around Asif lay flat on his chest on this concrete slab at the opposite side. I rushed to help him to get up; he was a bit shaken up but all right.

A few hours later Asif felt like he was passing urine, he knew that this was impossible as he had lost the ability to do so when his kidneys were taken out on his first trip to Pakistan. Instead he found blood trickling down into his underpants. Asif confided in me and did not want to upset Mum. When I saw the blood, I had to take a long deep breath. I felt as though something had struck me with a sharp object. I did not know what to do, and who to turn to. I could not ring 999 and get help as in back home! So I spoke to Akhtar and arranged to see Dr Zaman.

At the hospital the X-rays revealed nothing. To stop the bleeding, Dr Zaman gave Asif medication. After a few days the bleeding stopped.

Many days had passed since the incident, but Asif was still not his usual self. He lost his appetite and his colour was a bit off. I convinced Mum and Asif to return back to the UK, as things did not seem right with Asif's health.

By now we had been waiting in Pakistan for a kidney

transplant for two-and-a-half months. But the falling incident changed everything. We decided to leave without getting the kidney.

Chapter 9
Out of Luck

Back home Asif's luck did not improve, as events took a downwards spiral.

The hospital refused to treat Asif because he had travelled to Pakistan against their advice and taken risks to jeopardize his health further. Consequently Asif lost his dialysis place at the hospital where he was receiving treatment for years and which housed one of the country's biggest kidney units.

This was unusual, because the UK's National Health Service is a free for all facility. But apparently, in cases where the medical practitioners feel that the patient is risking his or her health unnecessarily, and is not fully cooperating to implement the plan of action for his or her wellbeing, the hospital has the right to refuse treatment. It came as a complete surprise to us.

Asif was given a place in a different hospital because he was a dialysis patient. Had he not required dialysis, he most probably would have had to pay for private treatment.

Months had passed and still Asif was not back to his usual self. He had not regained his appetite and was losing weight fast, but this was put down to the side effects of dialysis. Further X-rays did not show anything negative either.

I was visiting Mum and Asif at their house one day when Asif vomited blood. I called 999 and the ambulance took Asif into Accident and Emergency. He had suffered an internal bleed from a punctured lung and needed emergency surgery. Since haemodialysis patients are more vulnerable to falls, the cause of this could only be the incident in Pakistan.

Asif had a major operation to stop the bleeding but lost over half of his blood, which caused further complications. His body ached all over, his toes bent with pain and his eyes watered constantly. He could not lie down on the hospital bed – instead he curled up and did not have the energy to talk. Somehow, however, with sheer will power and determination he pulled through. His usual hospital agreed to resume all his treatment.

The dangers that we thought we had avoided now came to haunt us. As a result of sharing inadequately sterilised haemodialysis machines in Akhtar's clinic, Asif had contracted the hepatitis C virus. This diagnosis hit us like a ton of bricks falling on a glass roof. With the virus, another element was added to Asif's health problems. Not only did he face a limited life expectancy due to his kidneys, but also he would now have to contend with liver problems.

Asif was taken off the kidney donor list and advised that he would be put back on once the virus had been successfully treated. This could take years. Ironically what we had aimed to achieve through buying a kidney had totally and utterly backfired. At least for the foreseeable future Asif would continue his journey on dialysis. Though Asif strived for a better life by acquiring a kidney, even without one he never gave up on living, always full of hope.

In the years that followed, Asif developed heart failure, acute anaemia and respiratory problems. The hepatitis C virus progressed at a steady rate and three years after diagnosis, it began to affect his liver. Asif's case for being treated for hepatitis C was complicated as he was one of just a few patients in the world requiring this treatment whilst on haemodialysis. The doctors were unsure as to how the treatment would work, and awaited results from another patient in a similar situation before starting.

Nearly six years after Asif first made his fateful decision to purchase a kidney, his treatment for hepatitis C began. It was November 2012. This was to be a one-year course, during which Asif was to inject himself. The treatment had a lot of side effects, including severe depression. But Asif soldiered on. Over the next months there were early indications that his treatment was working.

In May 2013 Asif caught flu and was unable to shake it. After a week he was still unwell and his breathing was so heavy that I could hear it upstairs. On the day of his dialysis, Asif was unable to get to hospital by himself so I took him. He was out of breath from the short distance that he walked and was unable to carry on beyond the entrance. Asif was gulping for air; it was as if he had been jogging vigorously. I had to wheelchair him into the dialysis unit.

That same day he was diagnosed with pneumonia and admitted into the High Dependency Unit, where he had to wear an oxygen mask constantly to help him breathe. A day later he was transferred to the Intensive Care Unit as his lungs had deteriorated and he required one-to-one care.

Asif had assigned me and our younger sister, Shamin as his next of kin. He had been in hospital for just two days when he asked us to come in as the doctors wanted to talk to us. The doctors told us that most patients with the same rate of breathing as Asif only last a couple of days in that condition as they are soon overcome with exhaustion and pain of a burning sensation inside. They are then put on a ventilator to give them time to heal. Of those put on a ventilator, only 30% regain consciousness. I remember instantly bursting into tears. I feared the worst. Asif was so frail, yet I can still feel the strength of my brother's grip on my hand to comfort me.

Asif continued to fight, but on the tenth day he gave his consent to be put on the ventilator. Moments before he was put on the ventilating machine, with floods of tears, my elder brother, younger sister and I hugged, kissed and gave Asif our love as if he was going on a long journey. Although it was hard for him to speak, he pushed himself to say to my elder brother, 'You look after Mum.' We had to drag ourselves out of that room. It was agony.

Exactly three days later the medical team told us that after trying everything they were not able to help Asif, and he was only breathing because of the ventilator. On the evening of 30th May 2013, the ventilating machine was switched off and within 20 minutes, surrounded by all his family, Asif breathed his last breath and passed away with lung collapse and multiple organ failure.

Asif's last words still ring in my head. He was my mum's reason to be. Heartbroken, her pain was reflected in her eyes. Seven months later she too passed away, joining her beloved son.

Chapter 10
Hope for the Future

Perhaps my brother would still be alive had a kidney been available in the UK. Perhaps he would have lived longer had he not taken the risk of buying one from a developing country in his struggle to survive. It is too late for my brother but what about the rest who are still playing the waiting game?

We should at least consider other options to improve the lives of many and increase their life expectancy. To increase organ donor rates and curb the number of people who die while waiting for a kidney transplant.

We have to face this together, because this problem does not recognise any national borders, colour or creed. Chances are high that we may need it ourselves one day.

A system should be put in place which encourages people to donate their kidneys, both live and cadaver (after death). A system in which there is no room left for the black market kidney trade or criminal activity in organ trade, whereby the poor and vulnerable are the target and those in desperate need of a kidney are forced to take illegal steps.

The majority of kidney transplants are received from deceased donors, and although live donations have increased considerably over the years, more of these are required. Live kidney donations come largely from family members or friends donating to their loved one, but the number of non-directed altruistic organ donors continues to rise here in the UK. This is when someone is prepared to donate a kidney to an unknown individual who is waiting for a kidney transplant.

To increase live donations further and counteract the severe shortage of organ donation in the UK, it has been suggested that people should be paid to become live kidney donors – a system known as regulated paid provision. In which a legal organization is responsible for setting a fair price for compensation and regulating the arrangement. If some type of financial compensation is paid to donors it will give an incentive to more people to donate.

It could be argued that this paid provision system would appeal to mainly people from a poor background and lead to exploitation of the vulnerable. People who are on low incomes, have lost their jobs, or are in severe debt. Some may regret their decisions at a later date.

However, being poor does not mean you are incapable of making rational decisions and understanding the inherent risks associated with the choices you make. If someone wants to sell a kidney then it should be his or her choice – as long as he or she is aware of the risks involved. So many risks are taken by people in the pursuit of entertainment, hobbies, fulfilling their dreams, or for many other social and financial gains. This includes taking dangerous jobs such as in the armed forces, because they believe that the advantage outweighs the risks.

All around the world people take part in all sorts of medical research activities and are compensated for their time and risk. Many risk damaging their body for pleasure as in smoking, climbing mountains and skydiving. But ultimately it is their choice.

The human body is capable of operating efficiently on just one kidney. With modern scientific advancement in technology and medicine, the procedure of donating one kidney is safe.

The paid provision system put in place should have stringent regulations. Providing sufficient information so the donor is made aware of all the risks, their backgrounds are checked and a full assessment made before accepting their donation.

Another option to increase kidney donations legally and to stop the illegal trafficking around the world is to put a presumed consent policy in place. This can be either opt-in or opt-out. Currently the UK, like the United States, has an opt-in policy, which means you choose to become a donor whilst you are alive. In the UK you can do this by joining the NHS Organ Donor register.

In an opt-out policy, people can choose not to donate in their lifetime, but instead upon death, consent is presumed for organ donation. In countries where the opt-out policy is applied, an increase of up to 30% of organs could be available.

The presumed consent system would both increase the number of organs and kidneys available for donation and reduce any illegal activities in organ trafficking targeting Third World countries.

However, there is a problem with the presumed

consent policies for both the opt-in and opt-out options. Some families have succeeded in changing their deceased loved one's decision to donate. I have personally witnessed this happening when one of my school friends passed away suddenly and his family had his decision to donate overturned. I remember my father getting emotional when this family refused to donate the healthy organs right in front of him. He said that if this family – who were, incidentally, all doctors – were not able to save other lives by donating, what chance would there be for people like Asif?

My father was right. If educated families are unable to comprehend the benefit of donating to others, and fail to see the essence and goodness of the act, then we as a society have to open our eyes. How can our beliefs enable us to see other humans suffer? Religions teach us to protect the human race, so what makes us decide that we cannot give away a body part that no longer has any use to its owner?

It has become human nature to not do anything until disaster strikes. Until then, we sit in the audience, meekly looking on. Life is shaped by the choices we make. Not only can they affect those we love and the society we live in, but in the case of organ donation, they can reach the shores of far, faraway lands.

Please consider how your thoughts, words and actions regarding this most emotive topic can have on-going repercussions for other sons, brothers and beloved family members. Just like Asif.

#######

Return

I would crawl to the top of any mountain
Dive to the bottom of the ocean fountain

Walk through raging fire and burn
Oh! What I wouldn't do to have you return.

© Yasmin Ghurki

Disclaimer

While Kidney Research UK is keen to see more people join the Organ Donor Register, the Charity does not support any system of 'paid provision'.

Although we approve of compensating altruistic donors to ensure they are not disadvantaged as a result of their decision, we do not condone any scheme whereby people receive a monetary reward in exchange for an organ.

The decision to become a living organ donor is one which is extremely personal and should not be motivated, influenced or incentivized by the prospect of financial gain.

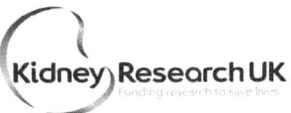

Acknowledgements

I would like to thank Stuart Wyle, Nicola Short and Peter Storey at Kidney Research UK for their full support.

My Mum, Dad and Asif, I thank you for everything. Rest in Peace. In our hearts you will go on.

A Note from Yasmin Ghurki

Thank you for reading this book. I hope that you liked it. I will be grateful if you could leave a review at your favourite online retailer.

I would love to hear from you, please contact me via:

Facebook: http://www.facebook.com/ghurki.yasmin

Twitter: http://YasminGhurki@GhurkiYasmin

www.ingramcontent.com/pod-product-compliance
Lightning Source LLC
Chambersburg PA
CBHW070552300426
44113CB00011B/1887